YOUR KNOWLEDGE HAS VALUE

- We will publish your bachelor's and master's thesis, essays and papers

- Your own eBook and book - sold worldwide in all relevant shops

- Earn money with each sale

Upload your text at www.GRIN.com and publish for free

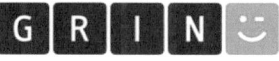

Bibliographic information published by the German National Library:

The German National Library lists this publication in the National Bibliography; detailed bibliographic data are available on the Internet at http://dnb.dnb.de .

This book is copyright material and must not be copied, reproduced, transferred, distributed, leased, licensed or publicly performed or used in any way except as specifically permitted in writing by the publishers, as allowed under the terms and conditions under which it was purchased or as strictly permitted by applicable copyright law. Any unauthorized distribution or use of this text may be a direct infringement of the author s and publisher s rights and those responsible may be liable in law accordingly.

Imprint:

Copyright © 2018 GRIN Verlag
Print and binding: Books on Demand GmbH, Norderstedt Germany
ISBN: 9783668631496

This book at GRIN:

https://www.grin.com/document/388765

Patrick Kimuyu

Mesenchymal Stem Cells as New Candidates for Stemcell Based Dental Therapies

GRIN Verlag

GRIN - Your knowledge has value

Since its foundation in 1998, GRIN has specialized in publishing academic texts by students, college teachers and other academics as e-book and printed book. The website www.grin.com is an ideal platform for presenting term papers, final papers, scientific essays, dissertations and specialist books.

Visit us on the internet:

http://www.grin.com/

http://www.facebook.com/grincom

http://www.twitter.com/grin_com

Mesenchymal Stem Cells as New Candidates for Stemcell Based Dental Therapies

Name: Patrick Kimuyu

Table of Contents

Introduction 3

Origin of Mesenchymal Stem Cells 3

Mesenchymal Stem Cells in the Dental Pulps and Oral Cavity 4

    Dental pulp DPSC 4

    Apical papilla SCAP 5

    Periodontal ligaments PDLSC 6

    Dental follicle DFPC 7

    SHED 7

    Gingival fibroblast GFSC 7

Therapeutic Mechanisms of Mesenchymal Stem Cells 8

Application of Mesenchymal Stem Cells in Dentistry and Dental Treatments 9

Conclusion 11

References 12

Introduction

Over the past few decades, stem cell research has gained extensive scientific inquiry. This aspect is attributable to the significance of stem cells in tissue engineering. It is apparent that tissue regeneration has emerged as a reliable medical approach for the treatment of tissue disorders and injuries (Wolf & Lamster 2011). Initially, embryonic stem cells were preferred as candidates for regenerative medicine because these cells can be induced to replicate in a pluripotent state (Estrela et al. 2011). However, stem cell research involving embryonic stem cells has attracted immense controversy. It is also associated with legal and ethical issues, thus limiting the use of embryonic stem cells in regenerative medicine (Hemmat, Lieberman & Most 2010). Fortunately, the discovery of mesenchymal stem cells (MSCs), also referred to as adult stem cells has restored promise for the development of stem cell therapies. Unlike embryonic stem cells, MSCs are free from legal and ethical concerns (Wei et al. 2013). MSCs are usually pluripotent progenitor cells that are generated in an array of tissues in both foetal and adult life. It is reported that these progenitor cells differentiate into cell types of the tissues that generate them, although studies indicate that they can differentiate cell types of other tissues (Meirelles Lda & Nardi 2009). Currently, MSCs are used for regenerative therapies for a number of tissue disorders and injuries including bone regeneration. For instance, MSCs generated by the dental pulps and the oral cavity tissues have been found to possess the potential for dental tissue regeneration (Estrela et al. 2011). These cells have also been found to useful in non-dental tissue repair (Demarco et al. 2011). Therefore, this paper will provide a comprehensive review on the origin and types of MSCs in the dental tissue and the oral cavity. It will also discuss their therapeutic mechanisms that make them useful in dentistry and dental treatments.

Origin of Mesenchymal Stem Cells

In retrospect, the origin of MSCs appears to be unclear with studies on the issue producing varying outcomes. Originally, MSCs were isolated from the bone marrow. However, recent research has identified other sources of MSCs including adipose tissue, endometrium, umbilical cord, peripheral blood, umbilical cord blood, periodontal ligament, dental pulp, placenta, and synovial membrane (Feng-Juan et al.2014). It is suggested that virtually all vascularized tissues in the body contain MSCs (Crisan, Yap & Casteilla 2008). Of special interest are the stem cells isolated from dental tissues. In 2000, dental pulp was discovered to have MSCs. Since then, different parts of immature and mature teeth have been identified as sources of MSCs including exfoliated deciduous teeth, human periodontal ligament, tooth germs, and the apical papilla (Estrela et al. 2011). MSCs from these sources have potential for multipotent differentiation, colony forming and self-renewal. Unlike bone-marrow-derived mesenchymal stem cells (BMMSC), stem cells from dental tissues have the capacity to differentiate into distinct cell lineages. It is suggested that MSCs from the dental and oral cavity tissues originate from the mesoderm and they constitute of non-haematopoietic stromal cells (Wei et al. 2013). Despite their mesodermic origin, their multipotency enables them to differentiate into mesodermic lineages, as well as endodermic and ectodermic cell lines (Salem & Thiemermann 2010).

Mesenchymal Stem Cells in the Dental Pulps and Oral Cavity

Oral cavity and dental tissues are known to generate an array of progenitor cells. For instance, dental mesenchyme, also known as the ectomesenchyme has stem cells with similar characteristics to those of the neural crest cells (Huang, Gronthos & Shi 2009). To date, five dental progenitor cells and two oral cavity-derived stem cells have been isolated. Human MSCs which have been isolated from dental tissues and characterized are dental pulp stem cells (DPSCs), stem cells from apical papilla (SCAP), periodontal ligament stem cells (PDLSCs), stem cells from human exfoliated deciduous teeth (SHED), and dental follicle progenitor cells (DFPCs) (Estrela et al. 2011). These progenitor cells are believed to be of odontogenic origin, thus they differentiate into odontogenic cell lines. However, studies indicate that dental-tissue-derived stem cells have the capacity for multilineage differentiation giving rise to other cell lines such as chondrogenic, myogenic, adipogenic, neurogenic, and osteogenic cells (Huang, Gronthos & Shi 2009). *In vitro* studies reaffirm that MSCs have trilineage capacity (Russell, Phinney & Lacey 2010). On the other hand, two MSC-like populations have been isolated from the gingival tissue: gingival fibroblast stem cells (GFSCs) and gingival epithelial stem cells (GESCs).

Dental pulp DPSC

Dental pulp stem cells (DPSCs) were the first to be isolated from adult dental tissue. These progenitor cells were found to reside in permanent third molars, primarily the root where they differentiate into odontoblast-like cells (Govindasamy et al. 2010). The key characteristics of odontoblast cells that differentiate from DPSCs include mineralization potential and active migration. As such, they are able to form three-dimensional dentin structures (Bakopoulou et al. 2011). Studies reveal variation in cell densities of DPSCs colonies. As such, it is apparent that the different cell clones exhibit varying growth rate. In addition, they exhibit variation in cell sizes and morphologies within the same colony. Biologically, it is believed that the differentiation of DPSCs into distinct cell lineages depends solely on biological factors in the microenvironment. Some of the factors in the local microenvironment that determine the programming of DPSCs into specific cell lineages include transcription factors, growth factors, signalling molecules, extracellular matrix protein, and receptor molecules.

From the perspective of dental tissue stem cell research, it has been found out that DPSCs have the potential to differentiate into multiple cell lineages. Studies show that reprogramming of DPSCs can generate corneal epithelial cells, osteoblasts, adipocytes, chondrocytes, odontoblasts, neurocytes, and myocytes (Warren et al. 2010). In addition, DPSCs can be reprogrammed to form induced pluripotent stem cells (iPSCs) (Yan et al. 2010). For instance, DPSCs are induced to differentiate into odontoblastic cell lines by dentin matrix protein 1 (DMP1). DMP1 is usually a non-collagen extracellular matrix protein that forms components of dentin (Almushayt et al. 2006). As such, it can be extracted for use in DPSCs reprogramming into odontoblast cells. This helps in forming dentin, especially over injured dental pulp tissue. In addition, studies show that fibroblast growth factor and transforming growth factor β1 (TGFβ1) in the microenvironment can induce DPSCs to differentiate into odontoblast cells (He et al. 2008).

Biologically, DPSCs play key functions in the dental pulps. Studies indicate that pulp tissue regeneration is facilitated by DPSCs. They are primarily involved in reparative dentin formation. In addition, dental pulp cells play other biological roles including providing innervations, nutrition and oxygen to the dental pulp that is usually covered by dentin. On the other hand, hard dentin plays a protective role in protecting dental pulp. As such, the integrity of tooth function and shape is associated to the dentin (Estrela et al. 2011).

Apical papilla SCAP

The second type of dental-tissue-derived MSCs resides in the apical papilla, the SCAP. Histologically, apical papilla forms the apex of developing permanent teeth. The anatomy of the dental tissue comprises of a cell-rich zone that separates the pulp from the apical papilla. However, SCAPs are found in the soft tissue embedding the apices developing teeth which is termed as the apical papilla (Sonoyama et al. 2008). Compared to DPSCs, SCAPs have a higher potential for differentiation. However, studies show that these progenitor cells express lower levels of melanoma-associated glycoprotein (MUC18), VEGF receptor 1 and matrix extracellular phosphoglycoprotein (MEPE). In addition, SCAPs exhibit some distinct characteristics from DPSCs and BMMSCs. For instance, studies have revealed that SCAPs express CD24 although the expression of this protein is impaired by osteogenic stimulation. Overall, apical papilla can be distinguished from dental pulp by the presence of the precursor tissue (Huang, Gronthos & Shi 2009). Biologically, apical papilla grows into the dental pulp. However, these parts possess cells which exhibit different characteristics. It is also suggested that SCAPs could be the precursor cells which are involved in the root dentin formation. This is so because; SCAPs have been found to have the potential of differentiating into odontoblast-like cells (Estrela et al. 2011).

Periodontal ligaments PDLSC

Periodontal ligament (PDL) acts as one of the most essential components of the dental tissue. Anatomically, this ligament underlies the alveolar bone and the cementum. It is believed that this space replaces the follicle area which exists around the growing tooth. However, this replacement occurs at different stages of tooth development. In this case, the replacement of the follicle by the periodontal ligament is observed to take place in bud and cap stages of tooth development. It then matures during the stage of tooth eruption, in order to prepare the emerging tooth for its biological functions, especially occlusal forces. Unlike the composition of the PDL in the early stages of tooth development, its mature stage is characterized by the formation of major collagen fibres. These fibres form the embedment in alveolar and the cementum. As such, they fill the PDL. From a biological approach, the development of the collagen fibres within the PDL occurs as one of the principal ways of adaptation of the dental tissue to its functions. In this case, the collagen fibres are organized into supportive structures with appropriates which enable the tooth to absorb the forces generated during chewing. On the other hand, dental tissues have been found to exhibit other adaptive characteristics, especially tooth integrity against injuries and diseases. One of these adaptive features is the existence of progenitor cells which have the potential to differentiate into an array of dental cell lineages. Studies indicate that stem cells from the PDL are capable of generating connective tissue cells, adipocytes and cementum-like cells of the dental tissue. Therefore, PDLSCs have been found to play key roles in the development of the cementum and the regeneration of the alveolar bone (Trubiani et al. 2008). As such, these cells help in maintaining the tooth root.

Dental follicle DFPC

The fourth type of stem cells from the human dental tissues is the dental follicle precursor cells (DFPCs). Dental follicle refers to a connective or ectomesenchymal tissue which surrounds the developing tooth. Precisely, dental follicle covers the developing tooth germ, especially the dental papilla and the enamel during the early developmental stages. In most cases, this tissue forms an integral component of the tooth germ before tooth eruption (Huang, Gronthos & Shi 2009). Studies show that the dental follicle contains stem cells which facilitate the development of the periodontium. It is apparent that the alveolar bone, PDL and the cementum form from DFPCs. In humans, DFPCs have been isolated from the third molars, and they are characterized by the formation of less adherent clonogenic colonies compared to other MSCs derived from human dental tissues. Another key biological characteristic of DFPCs is the potential for osteogenic differentiation. Moreover, DFPCs have been found to exhibit fibroblast-like morphology. They also express some of the main dental tissue factors including Notch-1, bone sialoprotein (BSP), nestin, fibroblast growth factor receptor 1-IIIC, and osteocalcin.

SHED

Finally, dental pulps have been found to host other self-renewing and pluripotent cells which have been termed as stem cells from human exfoliated deciduous teeth (SHED). Evidence from dental stem cell research indicates that *in vitro* induction of SHEDs facilitates bone formation and the development of dentin. On the other hand, SHEDs exhibit diverse characteristics *in vivo*. Some of the key *in vivo* characteristics which are exhibited by SHEDs include osteoinductive capacity, increased rates of proliferation and population doublings. It has also been found out that SHEDs have the ability to pulp-like complexes. It is also believed that stem cells from the human exfoliate deciduous teeth produce neurotrophic factors, and this implies that they can differentiate into non-dental mesenchymal cell populations (Estrela et al. 2011).

Gingival fibroblast GFSC

Human gingival tissues have also been found to be sources of MSCs. At present, two types of MSCs have been isolated and characterized. These gingival-derived stem cells include gingival fibroblast stem cells and gingival epithelial stem cells. Both types of MSCs reside in the human gingiva, the tissue that surrounds the tooth. In the past studies on gingival mesenchymal stem cells (GMSCs), it is apparent that these cells exhibit several characteristics that make them capable of self-renewal and multilineage differentiation. For instance, it is evident that GMSCs have the potential to form osteoblasts and adipocytes (Zhang et al. 2009).

Therapeutic Mechanisms of Mesenchymal Stem Cells

Over the past few decades, extensive dental stem cell research has shown the great potential of MSCs regenerative medicine. Foremost, stem cells derived from dental tissues have been used as candidates for regenerative medicine, especially for the development of MSC-based therapies. As a result, a number of regenerative therapies for dental and non-dental disorders have already been developed. However, it is worth noting that there are critical concerns surrounding the use of MSCs for therapeutic purposes. Some of the concerns which remain unsolved include the fate of MSCs after infusion, optimal dosage, appropriate routes of administration, and the appropriate time of engraftment (Karp & Leng Teo 2009).

From a therapeutic perspective, MSCs' potential in regenerative medicine is solely attributable to their biological characteristics, including their therapeutic mechanisms. One of the key factors related to the therapeutic mechanisms of MSC-based therapies in the MSC niche. MSC niche refers to a concept in stem cell research which describes the micro-environment which enable stem cells to retain their 'stemness' potential. This specialized micro-environment contains an array of biological factors which enable the cells to flourish. The roles of elements which are necessary for the MSCs to retain their 'stemness' include the prevention of MSCs from death, determining the fate of MSCs progeny and regulation of MSC proliferation (Jones & Wagers 2008). For instance, the micro-environment which is provided by the bone marrow acts as an MSC niche for haematopoietic stem cells (HSCs). Studies show that HSCs flourish in different niches: perivascular and endosteal niches which maintain their proliferation and quiescence, respectively. In addition, the perivascular niche is also believed to mediate circulation, thus facilitating the retention of HSCs' 'stemness.' Despite the inadequacy of information regarding the ideal niche for BMMSCs, some studies suggest that the perivascular region of the bone marrow acts the ideal niche for adipose-derived MSCs and BMMSCs (Huang, Gronthos & Shi 2009). Similarly, DPSCs in human dental tissues have been found to reside in a micro-environment which is described as a DPSC niche. DPSCs are usually localized in perineural sheath and perivascular regions.

Another principal feature of MSCs which is associated to their therapeutic mechanisms is homing efficiency. Clinical studies indicate that MSCs tend to migrate to damaged tissue sites. However, some cells get trapped in the lungs following intravenous administration (Lee et al. 2009).This phenomenon is associated with the activities of cell trafficking-related molecules in the body. Some of the main biological molecules which are involved in this process are matrix metalloproteinases, chemokines and adhesion proteins such as the vascular cell adhesion protein 1 (VCAM-1) and P-selectin (Wei et al. 2013).

It has also been found out that MSCs exhibit immunomodulation effects. Studies indicate that allogeneic MSCs express immunosuppressive effects. As such, allogeneic MSCs supplement autogeneic MSC sources in the body. It is also worth noting that xenogeneic MSCs are usually rejected by the host after regeneration. In addition, these cells have been found to be well-tolerated the recipient hosts. Therefore, immunomodulation of MSCs serves as one of the key factors which enhance their use for therapeutic purposes. DPSCs have also been found to exhibit immunomodulation effects. This aspect is attributable to their capacity to down-modulate some immune responses, especially those which are mediated by B-cells, T-cells, KN-cells, and dendritic cells. Over the past few years, extensive stem cell research has shown that other dental stem cells such as PDLSCs and SCAP exhibit immunosuppressive properties (Huang, Gronthos & Shi 2009). Overall, it is believed that the efficacy of MSCs depends on the micro-environments in damaged tissues (Wei et al. 2013).

Differentiation potential and production of trophic factors are the other factors which underlay therapeutic mechanisms of MSCs. Ordinarily; MSCs have the ability to differentiate along different cell lineages. As such, their multipotent potential enables them to be applicable in regenerative medicine, especially in tissue repair. On the other hand, MSCs have been found to be reliable sources of trophic factors. As such, they stimulate the production of growth factors in damaged sites, thus facilitating tissue regeneration. Some of the main trophic factors which are produced by MSCs include basic fibroblast growth factors (bFGF), IL-6, vascular endothelial growth factor (VEGF), CCL-2, and insulin-like growth factor-1 (IGF-1). These biological elements play critical roles in mediating angiogenesis, as well as, preventing programmed cell death. As such, the capacity of MSCs to produce trophic factors enhances their underlying therapeutic mechanisms (Wei et al. 2013).

Application of Mesenchymal Stem Cells in Dentistry and Dental Treatments

In the recent years, focus on regenerative medicine has shifted to the development of dental MSC-based therapies. Stem cells from the dental tissues and oral cavity are now being used for dentistry and dental treatments. Foremost, tooth tissue engineering seems to rely solely on the therapeutic mechanisms of stem cells derived from dental tissues. Following successful trials on tooth tissue regeneration, it is apparent that dental stem cells can be used for repairs of tooth tissues such as the pulp, dentin and PDL.

One of the most reliable dental stem cell-based dentistry approaches is the bio-tooth engineering. In the past decade, PDLSCs and SCAP have been used for tooth regeneration, especially the restoration of the dentition through dental implants. Researchers have been able to generate a bio-root with PDL tissues through the use of PDLSCs in combination with SCAP (Huang, Gronthos & Shi 2009).

Second, stem cells from dental tissues have been used for regeneration of periodontal defects. For instance, PDLSCs have now become the touchstone for repair of periodontal defects in dentistry. These cells are used to generate acellular allogeinic bone grafts which are used for tooth regeneration. In addition, PDLSCs are induced to prepare platelet-rich plasma (PRP) in patients with periodontal defects. From a clinical perspective, PRP has been found to play key biological roles tooth regeneration including the promotion of bone regeneration and the enhancement of periodontal healing (Huang, Gronthos & Shi 2009). As such, the use of PDLSCs in regeneration of periodontal defects has become one of the most reliable MSC-based regenerative periodontal therapies (Liu et al. 2008).

Overall, all stem cells from dental and gingival tissues have the potential for regenerative medicine. This is attributable to their therapeutic mechanisms. In addition, MSCs have gained immense acceptance in regenerative medicine because they are not associated with ethical and legal issues. In retrospect, different dental stem cells have been found to have different applications in tissue repair. For instance, DPSCs have been found to generate dentin-like structures *de novo* in the root canal. Studies indicate that DPSCs can serve as a means of pulp tissue preservation because of their ability to form vascularised structures which are similar to the human dentin (Huang et al. 2010). In addition, the use of DPSCs in the development of dental MSC-based therapies for endodontic diseases holds the promise for a breakthrough in the management and treatment of dental disorders. On the other hand, SCAPs have been found to be capable of producing odontoblasts which form the root dentin (Sonoyama et al. 2008). Over the years, studies have been showing the occurrence of apexogenesis in damaged immature permanent teeth. This phenomenon has been found to occur in cases of abscess or periodontitis (Chueh & Huang 2006). In this case, the apical papilla survives pulp necrosis due to the presence of SCAP in the periapical tissues (Lovelace et al. 2010). Therefore, it is apparent that SCAP have the potential for future applications in the treatment of endodontic infections due to their high proliferative potential. Similarly, other dental stem cells such as SHEDs and DFPCs have been found to have potential tubular dentin and periodontal regeneration, respectively (Estrela et al. 2011).

On the other hand, GMSCs hold promise for regenerative dentistry. For instance, human gingival fibroblasts (hGFs) have been found to be reliable sources of iPSCs which are expected to be used for regenerative dentistry (Yu et al. 2016). On the other hand, GESCs have the potential to form whole tooth. As such, they are used for whole-tooth bioengineering (Volponi, Kawasaki & Sharpe 2013). Overall, stem cells play critical biological roles in oral diseases (Jones & Klein 2013).

Conclusion

Conclusively, the discovery and isolation of dental MSCs is considered as a breakthrough in regenerative medicine. These stem cells have become candidates for regenerative medicine owing to their multifactorial potential. Some of the key characteristics which make MSCs from the dental and gingival tissues suitable for the development of MSC-based regenerative therapies for dental and non-dental diseases include multi-differentiation into distinct cell lineages, high rate of proliferation and high viability. In addition, the discovery of MSCs has attracted immense scientific inquiry owing to their widespread acceptance as sources of stem cells for MSC-based regenerative therapies. Therefore, future approaches in dentistry, especially in the treatment of dental diseases are expected to exploit the therapeutic potential of dental tissue stem cells, as well as, stem cells from the oral cavity. It is apparent that PDL tissue regeneration through the use of dental tissue MSCs holds the promise for the treatment of periodontal diseases. In addition, successful MSC-based regenerative therapies are expected to improve the existing dental implant therapies, thus transforming dentistry and the entire clinical practice.

References

Almushayt, A, Narayanan, K, Zaki, AE & George, A 2006, 'Dentin matrix protein 1 induces cytodifferentiation of dental pulp stem cells into odontoblasts', *Gene Therapy*, vol. 13, pp. 611-620.

Bakopoulou A, Leyhausen G, Volk J, Tsiftsoglou A, Garefis P,Koidis P, et al.. Comparative analysis of in vitro osteo/odontogenic differentiation potential of human dental pulp stem cells (DPSCs) and stem cells from the apical papilla (SCAP). *Arch Oral Biol.*, vol. 2010.12.008.

Chueh, LH & Huang, GT 2006, 'Immature teeth with periradicular periodontitis or abscess undergoing apexogenesis: a paradigm shift', *J Endod.*, vol. 32, pp. 1205-1213.

Crisan, M, Yap, S & Casteilla L 2008, 'A perivascular origin for mesenchymal stem cells in multiple human organs', *Cell Stem Cell*, vol. 3, pp. 301–313.

Demarco, FF, Conde, M, Cavalcanti, BN, Casagrande, L, Sakai, VT & Nör, JE 2011, 'Dental pulp tissue engineering', *Braz Dent J.*, vol. 22, pp. 3-14.

Estrela, C, Alencar, A, Kitten, G, Vencio, E & Gava, E 2011, 'Mesenchymal stem cells in the dental tissues: perspectives for tissue regeneration', *Braz Dent J.*, vol. 22 no. 2, pp. 91-98.

Feng-Juan, L, Tuan, R, Cheung, K & Leung, V2014, 'Concise review: the surface markers and identity of human mesenchymal stem cells', *Stem cells*, vol. 32, pp. 1408–1419.

Govindasamy, V, Abdullah, AN, Ronald, VS, Musa, S, Ab Aziz, ZA & Zain, RB 2010, 'Inherent differential propensity of dental pulp stem cells derived from human deciduous and permanent teeth', *J Endod.*, 36, pp. 1504-1515.

He, H, Yu, J, Liu, Y, Lu, S, Liu, H & Shi, J 2008, 'Effects of FGF2 and TGFbeta1 on the differentiation of human dental pulp stem cells in vitro', *Cell Biol Int.*, vol. 32, pp. 827-834.

Hemmat, S, Lieberman, DM & Most, SP 2010, 'An introduction to stem cell biology', *Facial Plast Surg.*, vol. 26, pp. 343-349.

Huang, GT, Gronthos, S & Shi, S 2009, 'Mesenchymal stem cells derived from dental tissues vs. those from other sources: their biology and role in regenerative medicine', *J Dent Res.*, vol. 88 no. 9, pp. 792–806.

Huang, GT, Yamaza, T, Shea, LD, Djouad, F, Kuhn, NZ & Tuan, RS 2010, 'Stem/progenitor cell-mediated de novo regeneration of dental pulp with newly deposited continuous layer of dentin in an in vivo model', *Tissue Eng Part A*, vol. 16, pp. 605-615.

Jones, DL & Wagers, AJ 2008, 'No place like home: anatomy and function of the stem cell niche', *Nat Rev Mol Cell Biol.*, vol. 9, pp. 11-21.

Jones, K, & Klein, O 2013, 'Oral epithelial stem cells in tissue maintenance and disease: the first steps in a long journey', *International Journal of Oral Science*, vol. 5, pp. 121–129.

Karp, JM & Leng Teo, GS 2009, 'Mesenchymal stem cell homing: the devil is in the details', *Cell Stem Cell*, vol. 4, pp. 206–16.

Lee, RH, Pulin, AA, Seo, MJ, Kota, DJ, Ylostalo, J & Larson, BL 2009, 'Intravenous hMSCs improve myocardial infarction in mice because cells embolized in lung are activated to secrete the anti-inflammatory protein TSG-6', *Cell Stem Cell*, vol. 5, pp. 54–63.

Liu, Y, Zheng, Y, Ding, G, Fang, D, Zhang, C & Bartold, PM, 2008, 'Periodontal ligament stem cell-mediated treatment for periodontitis in miniature swine, '*Stem Cells*, vol. 26, pp. 1065-1073.

Lovelace, TW, Henry, MA, Hargreaves, KM & Diogenes, A 2010, 'Evaluation of the delivery of mesenchymal stem cells into the root canal space of necrotic immature teeth after clinical regenerative endodontic procedure', *J Endod.*, vol. 37, pp. 133-138.

Meirelles LS & Nardi, NB 2009, 'Methodology, biology and clinical applications of mesenchymal stem cells', *Front Biosci.*, vol. 14, pp. 4281-4298.

Russell, KC, Phinney, DG & Lacey, MR 2010, 'In vitro high-capacity assay to quantify the clonal heterogeneity in trilineage potential of mesenchymal stem cells reveals a complex hierarchy of lineage commitment', *Stem Cells*, vol. 28, pp. 788–798.

Salem, HK & Thiemermann, C 2010, 'Mesenchymal stromal cells: current understanding and clinical status', *Stem Cells*, vol. 28, pp. 585–96.

Sonoyama, W, Liu, Y, Yamaza,T, Tuan, RS, Wang, S & Shi S 2008, 'Characterization of the apical papilla and its residing stem cells from human immature permanent teeth: a pilot study', *J Endod.*, vol. 34, pp. 166-171.

Trubiani, O, Orsini, G, Zini, N, Di Iorio, D, Piccirilli, M & Piattelli, A 2008, 'Regenerative potential of human periodontal ligament derived stem cells on three-dimensional biomaterials: a morphological report', *J Biomed Mater Res A*, vol. 87, pp. 986-993.

Volponi, A, Kawasaki, M & Sharpe, PT 2013, 'Adult human gingival epithelial cells as a source for whole-tooth bioengineering', *J Dent Res.*, 92 no.4, pp. 329-34.

Warren, L, Manos, PD, Ahfeldt, T, Loh, YH, Li, H & Lau, F 2010, 'Highly efficient reprogramming to pluripotency and directed differentiation of human cells with synthetic modified mRNA', *Cell Stem Cell*, vol. 7, pp. 618-630.

Wei, X, Yang, X, Han, Z, Qu, F, Shao, L & Shi, Y 2013, 'Mesenchymal stem cells: a new trend for cell therapy', *Acta Pharmacologica Sinica*, vol. 34, pp. 747–754.

Wolf, DL & Lamster, IB 2011, 'Contemporary concepts in the diagnosis of periodontal disease', *Dent Clin North Am.*, 55, pp. 47-61.

Yan, X, Qin, H, Qu, C, Tuan, RS, Shi, S & Huang, GT 2010, 'iPS cells reprogrammed from human mesenchymal-like stem/progenitor cells of dental tissue origin', *Stem Cells Dev.*, vol. 19, pp. 469-480.

Yu, G, Okawa, H, Okita, K, Kamano, Y, Wang, F, Saeki, M, Yatani, H & Equsa, H 2016, 'Gingival fibroblasts as autologous feeders for induced pluripotent stem cells', *J Dent Res.*, 95 no. 1, 110-8.

Zhang, Q, Shi, S, Liu, Y, Uyanne, J, Shi, Y, Shi, S & Le, A 2009, 'Mesenchymal stem cells derived from human gingiva are capable of immunomodulatory functions and ameliorate inflammation-related tissue destruction in experimental colitis', *J Immunol.*, vol. 183 no. 12, pp. 7787–7798.

YOUR KNOWLEDGE HAS VALUE

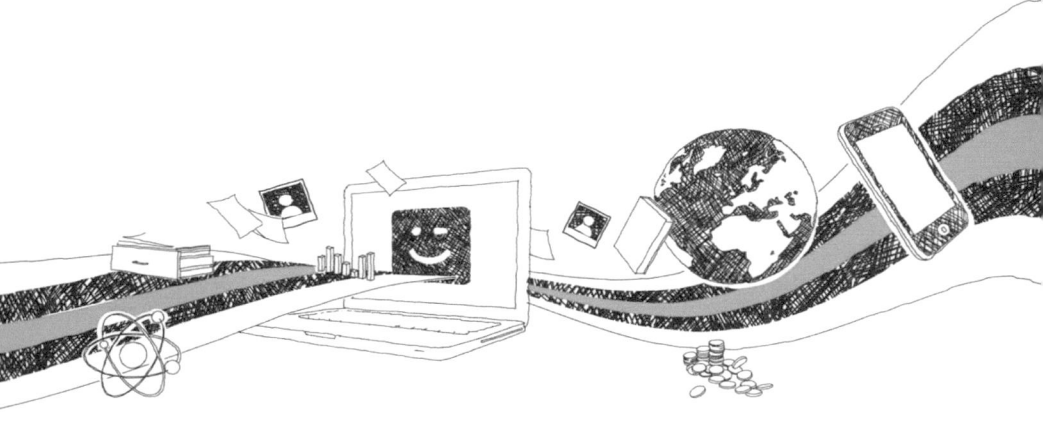

- We will publish your bachelor's and master's thesis, essays and papers

- Your own eBook and book - sold worldwide in all relevant shops

- Earn money with each sale

Upload your text at www.GRIN.com
and publish for free

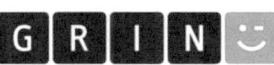